The Art of Hospice Visit Planning

The Art of Hospice Visit Planning

A Clinical Guide to Patient-Centered Care Frequency

Peter M. Abraham, BSN, RN

The Art of Hospice Visit Planning
A Clinical Guide to Patient-Centered Care Frequency
Copyright © 2024 Peter M. Abraham, BSN, RN

All rights reserved. No part of this book may be reproduced or transmitted in any manner whatsoever without written permission, except for brief quotations embodied in critical articles and reviews. This book is a work of nonfiction intended for educational purposes only.

This book is a work of non-fiction. The views expressed are solely those of the author and do not necessarily reflect the publisher's opinions, and the publisher disclaims any responsibility for them as a result.

Contact Info: author@2abraham.com

Dedication

This book is dedicated to all my fellow hospice nurses—yes, to you! Like me, you are out there every workday, caring for the terminally ill—those living in their darkest hours—and here you are, bringing light into their day. Special thanks to Stacey Rowse, RN, who introduced me to the Sunset Scale, discussed in this book as a tool to help determine hospice nurse visit frequencies.

Thank you to all my fellow hospice nurses!

Table of Contents

Introduction _____ *1*

    The Critical Role of Visit Frequency in Hospice Care _____ 2

    Impact on Patient Outcomes and Family Satisfaction _____ 4

    Overview of Current Challenges in Visit Planning _____ 5

Chapter 1: Fundamentals of Hospice Visit Planning _____ *8*

    Core Principles of Visit Frequency _____ 10

    Medicare Guidelines and Requirements _____ 12

    Basic Assessment Tools _____ 13

    Documentation Requirements _____ 15

    Conclusion to Chapter 1: Fundamentals of Hospice Visit Planning _____ 16

Chapter 2: Advanced Considerations for Visit Frequency ___ *19*

    Clinical Indicators for Frequency Adjustment _____ 20

    Palliative Performance Scale Assessment _____ 22

    Time-Based Visit Planning _____ 24

    Team Communication Strategies _____ 25

    Conclusion to Chapter 2: Advanced Considerations for Visit Frequency_ 26

Chapter 3: The Sunset Assessment Scale _____ *29*

    Understanding the Scale Components _____ 31

    Scoring Methodology _____ 32

Implementation Guidelines _____ 34

Case Studies and Examples _____ 36

Conclusion to Chapter 3: The Sunset Assessment Scale _____ 37

Chapter 4: Comparative Analysis of Assessment Methods __ 40

Traditional vs. Sunset Scale Approaches _____ 42

Strengths and Limitations _____ 43

Integration Strategies _____ 44

Best Practices for Implementation _____ 46

Conclusion to Chapter 4: Comparative Analysis of Assessment Methods 48

Chapter 5: Crisis Prevention Through Strategic PRN Planning 51

Identifying Potential Crisis Points _____ 52

Proactive Visit Planning _____ 54

Family Education and Support _____ 56

Documentation and Communication Protocols _____ 57

Conclusion to Chapter 5: Crisis Prevention Through Strategic PRN Planning
_____ 58

Conclusion _____ *61*

Call to Action for Excellence _____ 61

Future Directions in Visit Planning _____ 61

Resources for Continued Learning _____ 62

Quality Improvement Strategies _____ 62

*Resources and References*_____ *63*

*Author Bio*_____ *67*

Introduction

Achieving Enhanced Hospice Care Outcomes

Increase Family Satisfaction

Enhance family satisfaction by 25% with improved care planning.

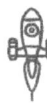

Fewer After-hours Calls

Reduce after-hours calls by 40% through proactive care.

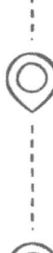

Reduce Readmissions

Decrease hospital readmissions by 30% with effective visit strategies.

CAHPS Scores

Improve patient feedback scores by 15-20% through better visit planning.

The foundation of exceptional hospice care rests upon thoughtfully planned nursing visit frequencies. As hospice clinicians, we ensure our patients receive the proper care at the right time. Visit frequency planning transcends basic scheduling – it's an art that combines clinical expertise, patient needs assessment, and resource management.

The Critical Role of Visit Frequency in Hospice Care

As hospice nurses and clinical managers, we understand that determining the right frequency of nursing visits is one of our most crucial responsibilities. Our decisions about when and how often to see our patients ripple through the entire spectrum of care, affecting the patient's comfort and symptom management, the family's peace of mind, and our organization's effectiveness.

Think back to your early days in hospice nursing. Perhaps you inherited a caseload where every patient was scheduled for weekly visits, regardless of their condition or needs. Or maybe you struggled with the uncertainty of whether you were visiting too often or not enough. These common experiences highlight why mastering visit frequency determination is vital to our practice.

Consider Mrs. Johnson, a typical hospice patient with end-stage COPD. When she first came onto service, her symptoms were well-controlled with routine medications, and she had strong family support. A standard weekly visit schedule seemed appropriate. However, as her disease progressed, subtle changes in her condition began to emerge. Her daughter started calling the on-call nurse more frequently, especially in the evenings, reporting increased anxiety and breathlessness. This scenario illustrates why static visit schedules often fail to meet our patients' evolving needs.

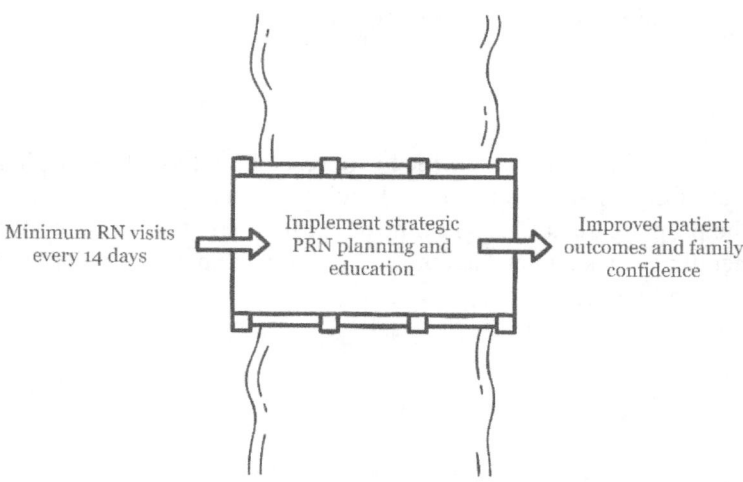

The art of determining visit frequencies requires us to think beyond the minimum Medicare requirement of one RN visit every 14 days. We must consider the dynamic nature of terminal illness, the capabilities of family caregivers, and the complex interplay of physical, emotional, and spiritual needs that characterize end-of-life care.

When we get visit frequencies right, we see remarkable outcomes. Patients experience better symptom management because we catch changes early. Families feel more supported and confident in their caregiving roles. Our on-call nurses receive fewer crisis calls, and our documentation reflects a proactive rather than reactive approach to care. Most importantly, we fulfill our promise to provide comprehensive, patient-centered hospice care.

However, determining appropriate visit frequencies isn't simply about increasing the number of visits when problems arise. It requires a sophisticated understanding of disease trajectories, assessment skills, and resource management. This book will explore the tools, frameworks, and clinical reasoning skills needed to master this essential aspect of hospice nursing.

Our journey together through these pages will transform how you approach visit planning. Whether you're a new hospice nurse seeking guidance or an experienced clinical manager looking to optimize your team's performance, the principles and strategies we'll discuss will enhance your ability to provide exceptional end-of-life care.

The art of visit frequency planning represents the intersection of clinical expertise, compassionate care, and operational excellence. As we delve deeper into this topic, you'll discover how mastering this skill can elevate your practice and, most importantly, improve the lives of our patients and families.

Impact on Patient Outcomes and Family Satisfaction

Clinical Impact

Patient outcomes significantly improve when we carefully plan our visit frequencies. Studies show that patients receiving well-planned hospice visits experience better pain control, with 80% of families reporting appropriate pain medicine administration. Similarly, patients receive more effective breathing support, with 78% of families reporting adequate relief of respiratory symptoms.

Consider Mrs. Rodriguez, who initially received routine weekly visits for her end-stage heart failure. When her nurse noticed subtle changes in her condition and increased the visit frequency, Mrs. Rodriguez's symptoms remained well-controlled, and her family felt more confident in providing care between visits.

Family Experience

The impact on families proves equally significant. Satisfaction rates increase markedly when visit frequencies align with patient and family needs. Families report higher confidence levels in providing care and experience less anxiety about their loved one's comfort.

More importantly, families whose loved ones receive appropriately timed visits report that end-of-life wishes were followed 80% of the time, compared to 74% when visit timing was less optimal. This difference might seem small, but it represents countless moments of peace and dignity during life's most challenging transition.

Quality Metrics

Strategic visit planning influences several key quality indicators:

Emergency Care Reduction

Proper visit frequency planning leads to the following:

- 40% fewer after-hours calls

- Reduced emergency department visits
- Fewer crisis situations requiring immediate intervention

Family Satisfaction

Well-planned visits result in the following:

- Higher CAHPS scores
- Improved pain management ratings
- Better symptom control reports
- Increased likelihood of recommending the hospice to others

The evidence clearly shows that thoughtfully planning our visit frequencies creates an environment where patients and families feel supported and cared for. This support translates into measurable improvements in clinical outcomes and family satisfaction, ultimately fulfilling our mission to provide exceptional end-of-life care.

Remember, each visit frequency decision we make has the potential to significantly impact a family's hospice experience. Understanding these impacts can help us better align our visit planning with optimal patient care and family support goals.

Overview of Current Challenges in Visit Planning

As hospice nurses and clinical managers, we face numerous challenges when planning patient visits. Understanding these challenges helps us develop better strategies to overcome them while maintaining high-quality patient care. The book *Mindful Minutes: Time Management Secrets for Hospice Nursing Excellence* explains how to overcome these challenges and spend more time with your patient and family without compromising your life-work balance.

Time Management Challenges

One of the most significant barriers we face is time management. Even with careful planning, our schedules can quickly become disrupted. A routine 45-minute visit might extend to three hours if a patient begins actively dying. We must balance these unpredictable situations while still meeting the needs of other patients on our schedule.

Consider Sarah, an experienced hospice nurse who typically sees five patients daily. Her carefully planned schedule changed dramatically when her second patient of the day showed signs of imminent death. While she needed to stay with this patient and family, she also had to coordinate with her team to ensure that her other patients received care.

Resource Constraints

Staffing shortages and geographic challenges significantly impact visit planning. Rural hospice nurses often travel 5-60 miles between visits, making it crucial to consider drive time when scheduling. Additionally, the limited availability of medications and transportation can affect our ability to provide timely care.

Communication Barriers

Effective communication remains a persistent challenge in hospice care. Families often misunderstand the purpose of visit frequencies, leading to unrealistic expectations. Some struggle with the concept of transitioning from curative to comfort care, affecting their receptiveness to our visit schedule recommendations.

Documentation Requirements

Medicare's increasing focus on quality metrics and documentation creates additional pressure on visit planning. We must ensure our visit frequencies meet patient needs and align with regulatory requirements while maintaining thorough documentation of care provided.

Complex Patient Needs

Each hospice patient presents unique challenges requiring individualized care planning. With an average of four unique problems per nursing visit, we must efficiently address multiple issues while maintaining the flexibility to adjust visit frequencies as conditions change.

The complexity of these challenges might seem overwhelming, but they also present opportunities for improvement. Through strategic planning, team collaboration, and patient-centered care approaches, we can develop visit schedules that better serve our patients while effectively meeting regulatory requirements and managing our resources.

Throughout this book, we'll explore practical solutions to these challenges, providing you with tools and strategies to optimize your visit planning process while maintaining the highest standards of hospice care.

Chapter 1: Fundamentals of Hospice Visit Planning

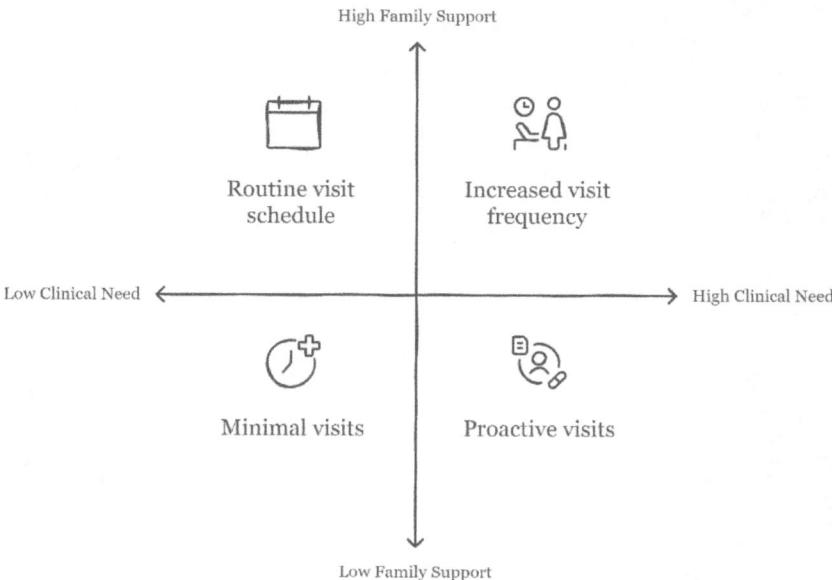

As we begin our journey into mastering hospice visit planning, let's consider why these fundamental concepts form the cornerstone of excellent hospice care. As a hospice nurse and a clinical manager, I've witnessed how proper visit planning transforms patient care, family satisfaction, and team efficiency.

I remember my early days in hospice, feeling overwhelmed by the responsibility of determining visit frequencies. Like many of you, I wondered: How often should I visit? What factors should guide my decisions? How do I document my rationale? These questions helped me better understand the fundamental principles in this chapter.

Learning Objectives

After completing this chapter, you will be able to:

- Apply core principles of visit frequency determination to your daily practice
- Navigate Medicare guidelines while maintaining patient-centered care
- Utilize basic assessment tools to support visit planning decisions
- Create comprehensive documentation that supports your clinical decisions

Key Concepts

The fundamentals of visit planning rest on four essential pillars. First, we'll explore the core principles that guide frequency decisions, understanding how patient needs, disease trajectories, and family dynamics influence our planning. Next, we'll navigate Medicare guidelines, learning to meet regulatory requirements while maintaining individualized care.

We'll then examine basic assessment tools that support our clinical decision-making. When properly utilized, these tools help us objectively evaluate patient needs and document our rationale for visit frequencies. Finally, we'll master the art of documentation, ensuring our notes tell the complete story of each patient's care journey.

Throughout this chapter, we'll share real-world examples and practical applications. You'll meet patients like Mr. Thompson, whose complex symptoms required frequent adjustment of visit schedules, and Mrs. Rodriguez, whose case demonstrates how proper documentation supports clinical decision-making.

Remember, mastering these fundamentals isn't just about meeting requirements—it's about providing the highest-quality care possible while effectively managing our valuable nursing resources. Let's begin this important journey together.

Core Principles of Visit Frequency

As hospice clinicians, we often ask, "How frequently should I visit this patient?" This seemingly simple question actually encompasses one of the most complex aspects of hospice nursing. The answer lies not in a one-size-fits-all approach but in understanding and applying core principles that guide our decision-making process.

Let me share a story about Maria, a hospice nurse with fifteen years of experience. One afternoon, she admitted Mr. Jackson, a 72-year-old with end-stage lung cancer. His symptoms were well-controlled, and his wife seemed capable and confident in providing care. Following her usual practice, Maria scheduled weekly visits. However, within days, the on-call nurse received multiple calls from Mrs. Jackson, anxious about her husband's breathing. This situation highlighted a crucial lesson: visit frequency decisions require more than just clinical assessment – they demand a deep understanding of patient and family needs.

Determining visit frequencies begins with recognizing that each patient's journey is unique. Think about your caseload. You likely have stable patients with weekly visits, others requiring multiple visits per week, and some needing daily support during periods of crisis. What drives these differences? Our understanding and application of core principles guide these crucial decisions.

Consider Mrs. Thompson, another patient on Maria's caseload. Initially stable with heart failure, she received routine weekly visits. However, Maria noticed subtle changes during one visit – slightly increased edema and mild confusion, and her daughter mentioned increased nighttime restlessness. Rather than waiting for these symptoms to escalate, Maria increased the visit frequency to twice weekly. This proactive approach prevented a crisis and provided the family with needed support during a period of decline.

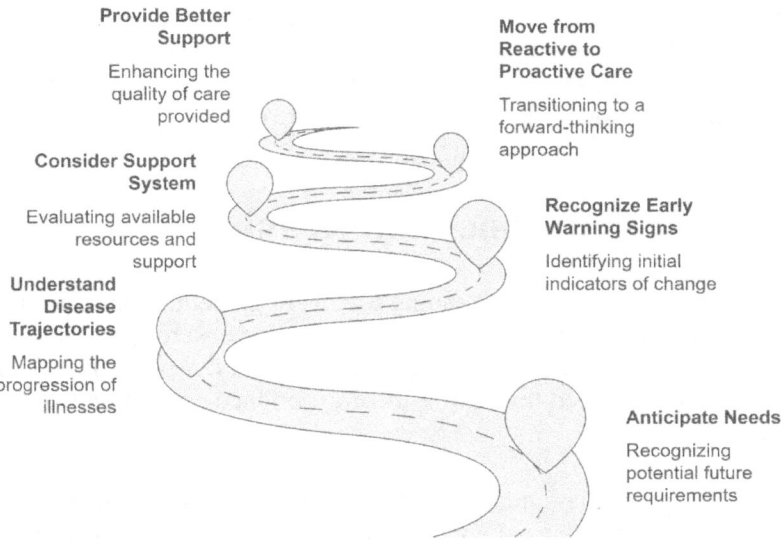

The foundation of visit frequency planning rests on our ability to anticipate needs before they become urgent. This requires us to understand disease trajectories, recognize early warning signs, and consider the entire support system available to our patients. When we master these principles, we move from reactive to proactive care, ultimately providing better support to our patients and families.

Experience has taught us that effective visit planning isn't just about clinical indicators. It's about understanding the family dynamics, cultural considerations, and support systems. Take Mr. Rodriguez, for example. His cancer was stable, but his wife's anxiety about caregiving meant more frequent visits were necessary initially. The visit frequency naturally decreased as her confidence grew through education and support.

As we continue this chapter, we'll explore how these core principles translate into practical applications. We'll discuss how to assess patient needs comprehensively, recognize patterns in disease progression, and make informed decisions about visit frequency that effectively serve our patients and our organizations.

11 | The Art of Hospice Visit Planning

Remember, mastering visit frequency determination is a journey, not a destination. Each patient teaches us something new, and each experience adds to our clinical wisdom. By understanding and applying these core principles, we can provide more effective, compassionate care while best using our valuable nursing resources.

Medicare Guidelines and Requirements

As hospice clinicians, understanding Medicare guidelines isn't just about compliance – it's about creating a framework that ensures our patients receive appropriate care while maintaining the integrity of our programs. Let me share what I've learned through years of experience navigating these requirements.

First, let's address the fundamental Medicare requirement that shapes our visit planning: every hospice patient must receive at least one registered nurse visit every 14 days. This isn't just a bureaucratic rule – it's a minimum standard to ensure quality care. However, as experienced hospice nurses know, most patients require far more frequent visits to maintain optimal comfort and support.

Consider my patient, Mr. Chen, who was admitted with end-stage COPD. While Medicare required only one visit every two weeks, his complex symptom management needs and his wife's anxiety about caregiving meant we initially scheduled visits three times weekly. As his symptoms stabilized and Mrs. Chen's confidence grew, we adjusted the frequency – but never fell below twice weekly visits, still well above the Medicare minimum.

Medicare's benefit periods also influence our visit planning strategy. Patients receive two 90-day benefit periods followed by unlimited 60-day periods. With each recertification, particularly as we approach the third benefit period, we must carefully document our visit frequencies to support continued eligibility.

A critical aspect of Medicare compliance is the face-to-face requirement. After the initial two 90-day periods, a hospice physician or nurse practitioner must conduct a face-to-face encounter no more than 30 days before each subsequent recertification. This requirement adds another layer to our visit planning, as we must coordinate these encounters with our routine nursing visits to ensure seamless care delivery.

Documentation plays a vital role in Medicare compliance. Each visit must clearly demonstrate the following:

- The patient's current condition
- Any changes in status
- The effectiveness of our interventions
- The rationale for our visit frequency decisions
- Plans for future visits

Remember, while Medicare sets minimum standards, our visit frequencies should always be driven by patient needs rather than regulatory minimums. As one of my mentors often said, "If you take care of the patient properly, the documentation will take care of itself." The key is balancing meeting regulatory requirements and providing individualized, patient-centered care. We can achieve both goals through thoughtful visit planning and thorough documentation while ensuring our patients receive the support they need throughout their hospice journey.

Basic Assessment Tools

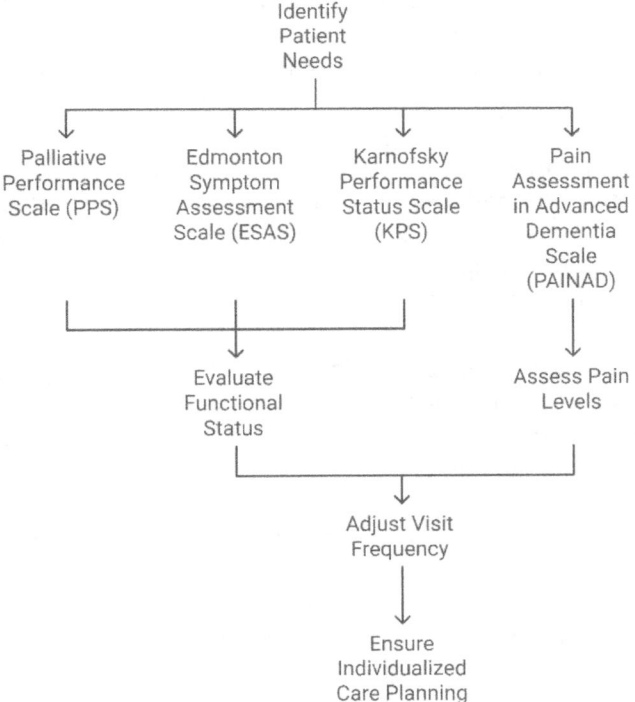

As hospice clinicians, reliable assessment tools help us make informed decisions about visit frequencies. Throughout my years in hospice care, I've found that combining several key assessment tools provides the most comprehensive picture of our patient's needs.

Let's start with the tools I've found most valuable in daily practice. The Palliative Performance Scale (PPS) has become my cornerstone assessment tool. I remember working with Mr. Johnson, a patient with end-stage lung cancer. His initial PPS score of 60% suggested he was still relatively independent but required occasional assistance. When his score dropped to 40% over three weeks, it signaled the need to increase our visit frequency from weekly to three times per week.

The Edmonton Symptom Assessment Scale (ESAS) is another invaluable tool in our arsenal. This nine-item assessment helps us track symptoms like pain, breathlessness, and anxiety. Mrs. Rodriguez's ESAS scores showed increasing anxiety and shortness of breath, prompting us to adjust our visit schedule before these symptoms became crisis situations.

The Pain Assessment in Advanced Dementia Scale (PAINAD) proves particularly useful for our patients with cognitive impairment. This tool helped me better assess Mrs. Smith's pain levels, even though she couldn't verbally communicate her discomfort. The resulting score guided our visit frequency decisions and pain management strategies.

The Karnofsky Performance Status Scale (KPS) offers another perspective on functional status. It provides a more complete picture of our patient's capabilities and needs when used alongside the PPS. I've found that tracking these scores over time helps identify subtle declines that might otherwise go unnoticed until they become emergent situations.

Remember, these tools aren't meant to replace our clinical judgment – they enhance it. By consistently using these assessments, we create an objective foundation for our visit frequency decisions while maintaining the art of individualized care planning.

Integrating these tools naturally into our assessments without visiting feels like a checklist exercise. Our patients and families appreciate thorough assessments but must feel heard and cared for. The data we gather helps support our clinical decisions and ensures we provide the right level of care at the right time.

Documentation Requirements

Throughout my years as a hospice nurse, I've learned that documentation isn't just about meeting regulatory requirements – it's about telling our patients' stories to support their care and ensure continuity across the care team. Let me share what I've discovered about effective hospice documentation.

Think about Mrs. Anderson, a patient with end-stage heart failure. When I first started caring for her, my documentation was basic: "Patient comfortable, no complaints." However, I quickly learned that such vague statements didn't serve anyone – not Mrs. Anderson, not the care team, and certainly not Medicare requirements. Instead, I began documenting specific observations that clearly depicted her condition and justified our visit frequency decisions.

Each visit note must be a comprehensive snapshot of our patient's condition. When documenting, we need to include the following:

- Specific changes in status since the last visit
- Effectiveness of current interventions
- Rationale for our visit frequency decisions
- Family education provided
- Plans for future visits

The art of documentation lies in being objective and specific. Rather than writing "slow decline," we should document measurable changes: "Patient's oral intake has decreased from 800ml to 400ml daily over the past week, requiring increased visit frequency to monitor for dehydration symptoms." Remember to document all aspects of care that influence visit frequency decisions. This includes:

- Phone calls and triage notes
- Family concerns and education needs
- Changes in symptoms or functional status
- Response to interventions

One particularly effective approach I've found is documenting at the bedside. This practice ensures accuracy and helps us capture subtle changes that might influence our visit frequency decisions. When I'm with a patient, I can document exact vital signs, pain levels, and symptom changes in real-time, providing a more accurate picture of their condition.

Our documentation should also reflect the dynamic nature of hospice care. When we change a patient's level of care or visit frequency, our documentation must clearly show when and why these changes occurred. This supports our clinical decisions and ensures continuity of care across the team.

Remember, good documentation tells a story that supports our visit frequency decisions while demonstrating the quality care we provide. It's not just about meeting requirements; it's about ensuring our patients receive the right care at the right time.

Conclusion to Chapter 1: Fundamentals of Hospice Visit Planning

As we conclude our exploration of hospice visit planning fundamentals, let's reflect on how these core concepts shape our daily practice. This chapter shows how understanding visit frequency principles, Medicare guidelines, assessment tools, and documentation requirements creates a framework for excellent patient care.

Key Takeaways

The art of visit planning requires us to balance multiple factors - from clinical needs to regulatory requirements, family dynamics, and resource management. Remember Mrs. Chen's case, where carefully applying these principles led to better symptom management and increased family confidence. Each component we've discussed is vital in ensuring our patients receive the right care at the right time.

Discussion Questions

1. How do you currently determine visit frequencies for your patients? What factors most influence your decisions?
2. Consider when you need to adjust a patient's visit frequency. What signs or symptoms prompted the change? How did you document your rationale?
3. Consider the assessment tools we discussed. Which do you find most helpful in your practice? How might you incorporate others to strengthen your visit planning process?
4. How does your documentation support your visit frequency decisions? What elements could you add to make your documentation more comprehensive?

Practice Scenarios

Scenario 1: The New Patient

Mr. Davis, 68, was newly admitted with end-stage COPD. He lives with his wife, who works part-time. No previous hospice experience. Oxygen-dependent, experiencing occasional dyspnea. Current medications include routine inhalers and PRN morphine for breathlessness.

- How would you plan initial visit frequencies?
- What assessment tools would you use?
- What documentation elements would you emphasize?

Scenario 2: The Changing Condition

Mrs. Rodriguez was on service for three months with end-stage heart failure. Previously stable on weekly visits, now showing increased edema, decreased appetite, and mild confusion. Family reports increasing anxiety at night.

- What changes would you make to visit frequency?
- How would you document the rationale for changes?
- What Medicare guidelines need consideration?

Scenario 3: The Complex Case

Mr. Thompson, advanced cancer with poorly controlled pain, lives alone with limited family support. Currently receiving twice-weekly visits but calling frequently between visits with concerns.

- How would you evaluate current visit frequency effectiveness?
- What documentation would support a change in frequency?
- Which assessment tools would be most valuable?

Moving Forward

As you continue your hospice nursing journey, remember that mastering visit planning takes time and experience. Each patient teaches us something new, and each challenge helps us grow as clinicians. The fundamentals we've covered in this chapter provide the foundation for the more advanced concepts we'll explore in the coming chapters.

Take time to reflect on your current practice. Consider how you incorporate these principles more effectively into your daily work. Share your insights with colleagues and learn from their experiences. Together, we can continue elevating the quality of hospice care we provide our patients and families.

Remember, excellence in visit planning isn't just about following guidelines - it's about combining our clinical expertise with thoughtful assessment and clear documentation to provide the best possible care for our patients and families.

Chapter 2: Advanced Considerations for Visit Frequency

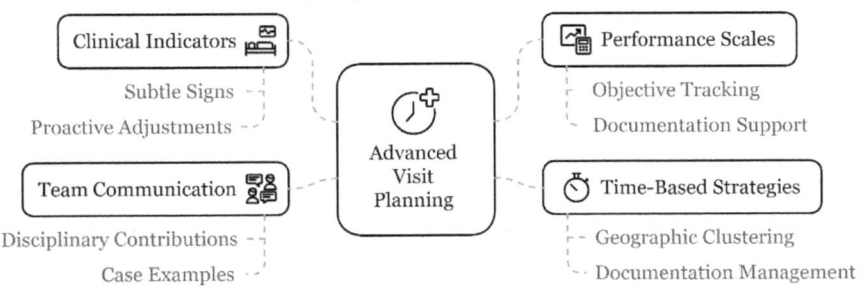

After mastering the fundamentals of visit planning, we're ready to delve deeper into the nuanced aspects that elevate our practice from good to exceptional. Throughout my years as a hospice nurse and clinical manager, I've discovered that understanding these advanced considerations often marks the difference between reactive and proactive care delivery.

I remember my early days in hospice when I relied primarily on noticeable clinical changes to adjust visit frequencies. Over time, I learned to recognize subtle indicators and patterns that, when properly interpreted, allowed me to anticipate and prevent crises rather than respond to them. This chapter will help you develop that same level of clinical sophistication.

Learning Objectives

After completing this chapter, you will be able to:

- Identify early clinical indicators that signal the need for visit frequency adjustments
- Apply performance scales effectively to support visit planning decisions
- Develop efficient time-based visit planning strategies
- Implement effective team communication protocols that enhance patient care

Key Concepts

Advanced visit planning builds upon four essential elements. First, we'll explore the subtle clinical indicators that often precede significant changes in patient condition. Understanding these early warning signs enables us to adjust visit frequencies proactively rather than reactively.

Next, we'll master using performance scales as objective tools for tracking patient status and justifying visit frequency decisions. You'll learn how these scales support clinical judgment and documentation requirements when properly utilized.

We'll then examine time-based visit planning strategies that help balance patient needs with practical considerations like geographic clustering and documentation management. Finally, we'll explore team communication strategies that ensure all disciplines contribute effectively to visit planning decisions.

Throughout this chapter, you'll meet patients like Mrs. Chen, whose case demonstrates how recognizing subtle changes led to timely visit frequency adjustments, and Mr. Thompson, whose care plan improved through effective team communication. These real-world examples will help you apply these advanced concepts in your daily practice.

Remember, mastering these advanced considerations isn't just about improving efficiency – it's about enhancing our ability to provide exceptional care while managing our resources effectively. Let's begin this next step in your professional development together.

Clinical Indicators for Frequency Adjustment

As hospice nurses, we often sense subtle changes in our patients that signal the need to adjust our visit frequencies. These intuitive observations and concrete clinical indicators guide our decisions to provide the right care at the right time.

Let me share a story about Mrs. Chen, a patient with end-stage COPD. Initially stable with twice-weekly visits, she began showing subtle changes – slightly increased anxiety in the evenings, minor changes in breathing patterns, and her daughter mentioned increased restlessness at night. These seemingly small changes prompted an increase in visit frequency to daily visits. This proactive approach prevented a crisis and supported the family during her final weeks.

Physical Indicators

When adjusting visit frequencies, several key physical changes deserve our attention. Patients transitioning toward end-of-life often demonstrate specific signs within three days of death, making this a critical period for increased support. These changes might include the following:

Breathing Pattern Changes

A shift in breathing patterns often signals the need for more frequent visits. Mrs. Rodriguez's case illustrates this ideally – when her breathing pattern changed from occasional dyspnea to regular episodes of breathlessness, we increased visits from weekly to three times per week.

Nutritional Changes

Declining oral intake often precedes other changes. We should consider increasing our presence when patients decrease their baseline intake to less than 500ml daily.

Support System Assessment

The strength of the patient's support system significantly influences visit frequency needs. Research shows that patients with strong family support and experienced caregivers often maintain stability with routine visits, while those with limited support may require more frequent nursing presence.

Disease Trajectory Considerations

Different terminal illnesses follow distinct patterns, requiring us to adjust our visit frequencies accordingly. For example, cancer patients often maintain relatively stable function until a precipitous decline in the final weeks, while heart failure patients typically experience a gradual decline punctuated by acute episodes.

Remember, our goal isn't just to meet Medicare's minimum requirement of one visit every 14 days – it's to provide comprehensive, anticipatory care that prevents crises and supports both patient and family through this journey. By carefully observing these clinical indicators and adjusting our visit frequencies accordingly, we create a care plan that truly serves our patients' evolving needs.

Palliative Performance Scale Assessment

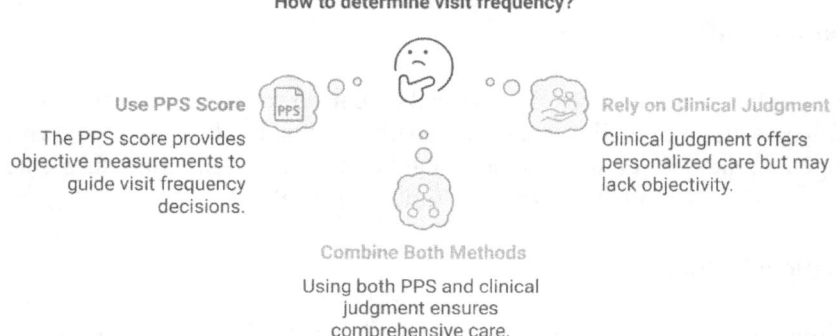

How to determine visit frequency?

Use PPS Score
The PPS score provides objective measurements to guide visit frequency decisions.

Rely on Clinical Judgment
Clinical judgment offers personalized care but may lack objectivity.

Combine Both Methods
Using both PPS and clinical judgment ensures comprehensive care.

The Palliative Performance Scale is one of the most valuable tools in our hospice nursing toolkit. I've found this assessment invaluable in guiding visit frequency decisions throughout my years in hospice care. Let me share how this tool has transformed my practice and can enhance yours. I remember working with Mr. Thompson, newly admitted with end-stage liver disease. His initial Palliative Performance Scale (PPS) score was 60% - he was still ambulatory but required occasional assistance. Within two weeks, his score dropped to 40%. This decline wasn't immediately obvious to his family, who saw him daily. Still, the PPS helped me objectively document the change and justify increasing our visit frequency from weekly to three times per week.

The beauty of performance scales lies in their objectivity. While our clinical judgment is crucial, having concrete measurements helps us communicate changes to families, team members, and insurance providers. Let's explore how to use these tools effectively.

Understanding Performance Scales

The PPS measures five key areas:

- Ambulation
- Activity level and evidence of disease
- Self-care abilities
- Oral intake
- Level of consciousness

For example, when I assess Mrs. Davis, I'm not just noting that she "seems weaker." Instead, I observe that she's transitioned from independent ambulation to requiring assistance with transfers, dropping from PPS 50% to 30%. This change signals a need to reassess our visit frequency.

Timing Your Assessments

Performance scale assessments shouldn't be limited to certification periods. I've learned to incorporate brief assessments during every visit, looking for subtle changes that might indicate declining function. This approach helped me identify Mr. Rodriguez's early decline, allowing us to adjust his care plan before a crisis developed.

Remember, these scales serve as tools to support our clinical judgment, not replace it. When Mrs. Chen's PPS score remained stable at 40%, but her anxiety increased significantly, we still increased visit frequency based on her emotional needs rather than physical decline.

The key is using performance scales as part of our comprehensive assessment. They provide objective data to support our visit frequency decisions while helping us track subtle changes that might otherwise go unnoticed. By mastering these tools, we enhance our ability to provide proactive rather than reactive care.

Think of performance scales as your clinical compass. They help guide your decisions while validating your clinical observations. When combined with other assessment tools and your clinical expertise, they become powerful allies in determining appropriate visit frequencies.

Time-Based Visit Planning

Understanding how to plan visits based on time considerations effectively is crucial for providing excellent hospice care while maintaining a manageable schedule. Throughout my years as a hospice nurse, I've learned that successful time-based visit planning requires structure and flexibility.

Let me share how I learned this lesson the hard way. Early in my career, I scheduled all my visits without considering the day's natural flow. I'd drive back and forth across town, arrive at patients' homes at inconvenient times, and struggle to complete documentation. Then, a mentor taught me a better way.

Strategic Scheduling

The most effective approach starts with planning your week before it begins. I recommend scheduling more complex visits early in the week and earlier when your energy levels are highest. Save time later in the week for unexpected follow-up visits or new admissions that inevitably arise. Consider Mrs. Johnson's case. As a high-acuity patient with complex symptoms, I scheduled her visits for Tuesday mornings. This allowed me to spend the necessary time with her while ensuring I had the mental clarity to manage her care effectively. It also meant if her condition changed, I had the flexibility to come later in the week.

Geographic Optimization

One of the most valuable lessons I've learned is the importance of grouping patients by geographic area. This isn't just about saving drive time – it's about being able to provide more consistent care. When patients in the same area are scheduled together, you can more easily adjust your timing if one patient needs extra attention without disrupting your entire day.

Documentation Management

Time management extends beyond visit scheduling. Documentation is critical and time-consuming. I've found the most successful approach is to complete documentation at the time of care, setting up a mobile office in your car with the necessary supplies and forms. This prevents the overwhelming pile-up of paperwork at the end of the day.

Remember, effective time-based visit planning isn't about rushing through visits – it's about creating a structure that allows you to be fully present with each patient while managing your overall caseload efficiently. When we master this balance, our patients and we benefit from more organized and effective care delivery.

Team Communication Strategies

Effective team communication forms the backbone of successful visit planning in hospice care. Throughout my career, I've learned that the most substantial patient outcomes emerge when the interdisciplinary team maintains clear, consistent communication channels.

Let me share an experience that transformed my understanding of team communication. We had a patient, Mr. Rodriguez, whose symptoms seemed stable during my visits, but our hospice aide noticed subtle changes in his appetite and energy levels during her more frequent visits. Because we had established strong communication practices, she felt comfortable sharing these observations immediately. This early warning allowed us to adjust our visit frequencies proactively, preventing a potential crisis.

Structured Team Meetings

Weekly interdisciplinary team meetings are our primary forum for discussing visit frequencies and care planning. Each team member brings unique insights about the patient's condition and needs during these meetings. Our social worker might notice family dynamics affecting care delivery, while our chaplain might observe spiritual distress requiring additional support – all factors influencing visit frequency decisions.

Real-Time Communication

Between formal meetings, immediate communication needs arise constantly. I've found that establishing clear protocols for urgent versus non-urgent communications helps maintain efficiency. When Mrs. Chen's daughter called reporting increased anxiety, our team's quick communication allowed us to coordinate an immediate nursing visit while scheduling follow-up support from our chaplain.

Documentation as Communication

Clear, thorough documentation serves as a crucial communication tool. When adjusting visit frequencies, I ensure my documentation clearly explains the following:

- The reason for the change
- Specific observations supporting the decision
- The new visit plan
- Expected outcomes
- Family response to the changes

Building Team Trust

The most effective communication happens when team members trust each other. This trust develops through:

- Consistent follow-through on commitments
- Acknowledgment of each team member's expertise
- Open sharing of concerns and observations
- Mutual support during challenging situations

Remember, effective team communication isn't just about sharing information – it's about creating a collaborative environment where every team member feels valued and heard. When we achieve this, our visit planning becomes more responsive and our patient care more comprehensive.

Conclusion to Chapter 2: Advanced Considerations for Visit Frequency

As we conclude our exploration of advanced visit frequency considerations, let's reflect on how these sophisticated concepts enhance our ability to provide exceptional hospice care. This chapter shows how combining clinical indicators, performance scales, time management, and team communication creates a comprehensive approach to visit planning.

Key Takeaways

The art of advanced visit planning requires us to synthesize multiple sources of information while maintaining efficiency. Remember Mrs. Rodriguez's case, where early recognition of subtle changes and effective team communication prevented a crisis and supported her family through a challenging transition. Each component we've discussed contributes to our ability to provide proactive rather than reactive care.

Discussion Questions

1. Think about a time when you noticed subtle changes in a patient's condition. What indicators led you to adjust visit frequencies? How did your team support this decision?
2. How do you currently balance time-based planning with the unpredictable nature of hospice care? What strategies have proven most effective?
3. Consider your team's communication patterns. What works well? Where do you see opportunities for improvement?
4. How has your use of performance scales evolved throughout your practice? How do they influence your visit frequency decisions?

Practice Scenarios

Scenario 1: The Subtle Decline

Mrs. Anderson, on service for two months with end-stage heart failure, is currently receiving weekly visits. Her daughter reports increasing fatigue and decreased appetite over the past week. PPS has dropped from 50% to 40%. She lives with her husband, who works part-time.

- What clinical indicators would you assess?
- How would you adjust visit frequencies?
- What team communication strategies would you implement?

Scenario 2: The Complex Schedule

You've inherited a caseload of 12 patients spread across three counties. Three patients require twice-weekly visits, while others receive weekly or biweekly visits. Two patients show signs of declining.

- How would you approach time-based planning?
- What factors would influence your scheduling decisions?
- How would you coordinate with team members?

Scenario 3: The Communication Challenge

Mr. Thompson receives nursing visits twice weekly. The hospice aide reports subtle changes during daily visits, but this information isn't consistently reaching the entire team. His wife seems increasingly anxious.

- What communication strategies would you implement?
- How would you ensure timely information sharing?
- What visit frequency adjustments might be needed?

Moving Forward

As you integrate these advanced concepts into your practice, remember that mastery comes through experience and reflection. Each patient situation offers opportunities to refine your skills in recognizing clinical indicators, applying performance scales, managing time effectively, and fostering team communication.

Take time to evaluate your current practices. Consider how to incorporate these advanced strategies more effectively into your daily work. Share your insights with colleagues and learn from their experiences. Remember, excellence in hospice care requires continuous growth and adaptation.

The skills we've explored in this chapter will serve as building blocks for even more sophisticated aspects of visit planning, which we'll discuss in upcoming chapters. Continue to observe, learn, and grow in your practice, always keeping our ultimate goal in mind: providing the best possible care for our patients and families.

Chapter 3: The Sunset Assessment Scale

Sunset Assessment Scale

Score	Activity	Nutrition	Body	Breathing
4	Alert/Interactive	2+ meals/day	Warm	Normal
3	↓ activity	Partial meals/tube	Feel cool	↑ effort
2	↑ hrs of sleep	Snacks or bites	Hands/feet cool	Short pauses
1	Sleep > 18hrs	Only drink	Hands/feet color	Long pauses
0	Min/No response	No Intake	Cold + color	Mouth open/shallow

Intuition: If anything seems off and you feel it suggests decline, and it is not reflected on this scale, deduct 2 points from the total score.

Scale: 12-16 No action   **8-12** Notify Office   **<8** ↑ visit freq.

Throughout my career in hospice care, I've searched for reliable tools to support visit frequency decisions. The Sunset Assessment Scale emerged as a game-changer, transforming how I approach patient assessment and visit planning. This chapter explores this innovative tool that combines clinical expertise with objective measurements to enhance our decision-making process.

I was initially skeptical about adding another assessment tool to our already busy days. Then, I met Mr. Thompson, whose subtle decline might have gone unnoticed without this systematic approach. His case, like many others we'll discuss, demonstrated how this scale could validate our clinical judgment while providing clear documentation support for our visit frequency decisions.

Learning Objectives

After completing this chapter, you will be able to:

- Apply the four core components of the Sunset Assessment Scale in patient evaluations
- Calculate and interpret scale scores accurately
- Implement the scale effectively within your practice
- Use case studies to guide clinical decision-making
- Document assessments that support visit frequency changes

Key Concepts

The Sunset Assessment Scale builds upon four fundamental elements that, when combined, provide a comprehensive picture of our patients' conditions and needs. We'll begin by exploring these components—activity, nutrition, temperature, and breathing patterns—and understanding how each contributes to our overall assessment.

Next, we'll master the scoring methodology that transforms our observations into actionable data. You'll learn how to assign appropriate scores and use the clinical judgment modifier to capture concerns that might not fit neatly into the standard components.

We'll then examine practical implementation guidelines to ensure you can integrate this tool smoothly into your daily practice. Finally, we'll explore real-world case studies demonstrating how the scale enhances our ability to provide proactive, patient-centered care.

Throughout this chapter, you'll meet patients like Mrs. Rodriguez, whose gradual decline was caught early through systematic assessment, and Mrs. Chen, whose case illustrates the importance of combining objective scores with clinical judgment. These examples will help you apply the scale effectively in your practice.

Remember, this scale isn't meant to replace your clinical expertise – it's designed to enhance it, providing structure for your assessments while supporting your visit frequency decisions with objective data. Let's begin our exploration of this valuable tool together.

Understanding the Scale Components

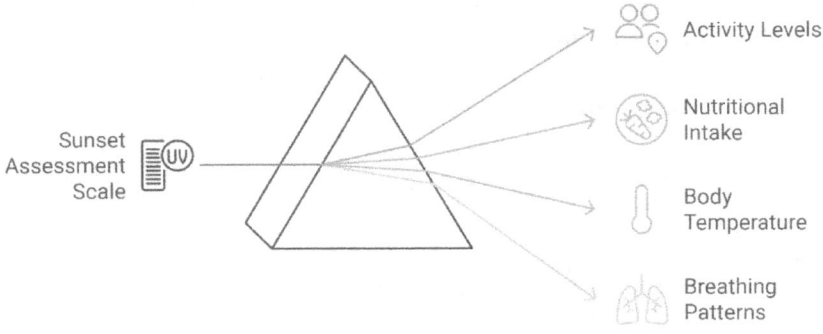

Throughout my years in hospice care, I've used many assessment tools, but the Sunset Assessment Scale has proven to be one of the most valuable for determining visit frequencies. Let me share why this tool has become such an essential part of my practice.

The Sunset Assessment Scale examines four critical areas that comprehensively picture our patients' conditions. Think of these components as pieces of a puzzle that, when assembled, reveal the full story of our patients' needs.

Activity Assessment

The first component measures activity levels. I remember Mrs. Thompson, whose gradual shift from independent movement to requiring assistance with basic activities signaled a need for increased visit frequencies. This component helps us track these subtle changes systematically rather than relying solely on general observations.

Daily Nutritional Intake

Nutritional intake often tells us more than just how much a patient is eating. When Mr. Rodriguez's intake decreased from regular meals to just sips of water, this scale component helped me objectively document the change and adjust our visit pattern accordingly.

Body Temperature

Temperature patterns can be surprisingly revealing. I've learned that subtle changes in body temperature often precede a more noticeable decline. This component helps us catch these changes early, allowing for proactive rather than reactive care adjustments.

Breathing Pattern and Effort

The fourth component assesses breathing patterns and effort. This isn't just about counting respirations – it's about understanding the quality and effort of each breath. Mrs. Chen's case taught me how valuable this component could be when her breathing pattern subtly changed before any other obvious signs of decline appeared.

Each component is scored from zero to four, creating a possible total score range from zero to sixteen. The beauty of this system lies in its simplicity and comprehensiveness. When we notice something concerning that isn't captured by these four areas, we can deduct two points from the total score, ensuring our clinical judgment remains part of the assessment process.

Remember, this scale isn't meant to replace our clinical judgment – it's designed to enhance it, providing objective support for our visit frequency decisions while ensuring we capture the complete picture of our patients' needs.

Scoring Methodology

The art of scoring the Sunset Assessment Scale effectively transformed my hospice practice, and I'm excited to share how it can enhance yours. Let me walk you through the process that has helped me make more confident, objective decisions about visit frequencies.

I remember feeling overwhelmed when I first encountered the scale's scoring system. Then, I met Mrs. Davis, a patient with end-stage COPD. Her case helped me understand how this systematic approach to scoring could validate my clinical observations and support my visit planning decisions.

Understanding the Scoring Range

Each scale component – activity, nutrition, temperature, and breathing – receives a score from zero to four. A score of four indicates optimal function, while zero suggests a significant decline. Let me share how this played out with Mrs. Davis:

When she first came onto service, her activity level earned a four – she was still independently mobile around her home. Her nutritional intake scored a three – she ate most meals but had started declining desserts. Her temperature patterns and breathing effort both scored fours. This initial total score of 15 supported our decision for weekly visits.

Tracking Changes Over Time

The real value of the scoring system emerges when we track changes over time. Two weeks later, Mrs. Davis's activity level dropped to a three – she needed occasional assistance with walking. Her nutritional intake remained stable at three, but her breathing effort decreased to three due to increased shortness of breath with activity. This decline in total score from 15 to 13 prompted us to increase visit frequency to twice weekly.

Clinical Judgment Modifier

One of the most valuable aspects of this scoring system is the clinical judgment modifier. When we observe concerning changes that aren't fully captured by the four main components, we can deduct up to two points from the total score. I used this with Mr. Thompson when his anxiety increased significantly, though his physical symptoms remained stable. This adjustment helped justify increasing visit frequency despite stable physical scores.

Remember, these scores should guide our decisions, not dictate them. They provide objective support for our clinical judgment while helping us communicate our reasoning to team members and document our decisions effectively.

The key to successful scoring lies in consistency and attention to detail. Each assessment should be thorough, considering obvious and subtle changes in each component. When we master this methodology, we enhance our ability to provide proactive, patient-centered care.

Implementation Guidelines

Implementing the Sunset Assessment Scale effectively requires a thoughtful, systematic approach. Throughout my years of hospice practice, I've learned that successful implementation depends on more than understanding the scoring system—it requires a commitment to consistent application and clear communication.

Initial Implementation

When introducing the Sunset Assessment Scale into your practice, start with a single patient. I remember implementing it with Mrs. Thompson, who had end-stage heart failure. By focusing on one patient initially, I could perfect my assessment technique and documentation before expanding its use across my entire caseload.

Routine Assessment Schedule

The scale works best when integrated into your regular visit routine. During each visit, assess all four components systematically:

- Begin with activity observation
- Progress to nutritional intake assessment
- Check temperature patterns
- Conclude with breathing pattern evaluation

Documentation Practices

Clear documentation proves essential for effective implementation. When I document my assessments, I include:

- Individual scores for each component
- Total score calculation
- Any clinical observations leading to point deductions
- Planned changes in visit frequency based on scores

Score-Based Actions

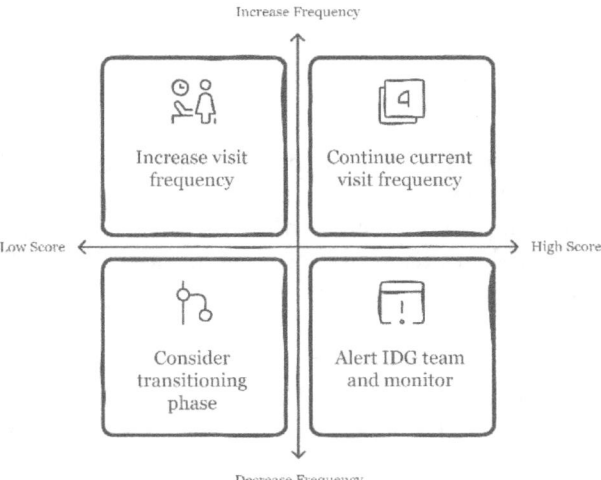

Hospice Visit Frequency Decision Matrix

The scale provides clear guidelines for action based on total scores:

- Scores 12-16: Continue current visit frequency
- Scores 8-12: Alert the IDG team and monitor for changes
- Scores below 8: Increase visit frequency
- Scores 0-4: Consider transitioning phase
- Score of 0: Consider imminent death

Team Integration

Remember that this scale serves as a guide to enhance, not replace, our clinical judgment. When implementing the scale, ensure all team members understand its purpose and application. Share your findings during IDG meetings and use the scores to support your visit frequency recommendations.

The beauty of this implementation approach lies in its flexibility. The scale adapts to any organizational setting while providing consistent guidance for visit frequency decisions. As you become more comfortable with the tool, it naturally enhances your clinical decision-making process.

Case Studies and Examples

Let me share some real-world examples demonstrating how the Sunset Assessment Scale transforms our approach to visit planning. Throughout my career, these cases have helped me understand the practical application of this valuable tool.

The Gradual Decline

Mrs. Rodriguez's case particularly stands out in my memory. A 78-year-old with end-stage COPD, she initially scored 16 on the scale – fully mobile, eating well, stable temperature, and comfortable breathing with supplemental oxygen. We scheduled weekly visits based on this assessment. Over three weeks, her scores told an important story:

Week 1: Score 16 - Weekly visits
Week 2: Score 14 - Slight decrease in activity level
Week 3: Score 11 - Notable changes in breathing patterns and reduced appetite

Because we tracked these changes systematically, we increased visit frequency before a crisis developed. The family later expressed gratitude for this proactive approach.

The Rapid Change

Mr. Thompson's case demonstrated how quickly conditions can change. His initial score of 13 supported twice-weekly visits. During one routine visit, I noticed significant changes:

- Activity score dropped from 3 to 1
- Nutritional intake decreased from 3 to 1
- Temperature patterns remained stable at 3
- Breathing effort declined from 3 to 1

His total score dropped to 6, prompting an immediate increase in daily visits. This quick response helped manage his symptoms effectively during his final days.

The Complex Situation

Mrs. Chen's case illustrates the importance of the clinical judgment modifier. Her physical scores remained relatively stable at 12, but her increasing anxiety and family dynamics weren't captured in the standard components. I deducted two points using the clinical judgment modifier, bringing her score to 10. This adjustment supported increasing visits to three times weekly, which helped address both her physical and emotional needs.

The Stabilization Success

Not all declining scores continue downward. Mr. Davis initially scored 9, requiring three visits weekly. His scores improved to 13 over two weeks through effective symptom management and family education. The objective nature of the scale helped us document this improvement and adjust visit frequencies appropriately while maintaining close monitoring.

These cases demonstrate how the Sunset Assessment Scale guides our clinical decision-making while remaining flexible to accommodate individual patient needs. Remember, each case teaches us something new about applying this tool effectively in our practice.

The key lesson from these examples is that the scale works best when combined with our clinical expertise and understanding of each patient's unique situation. It provides structure for our assessments while allowing room for professional judgment in our visit planning decisions.

Conclusion to Chapter 3: The Sunset Assessment Scale

As we conclude our exploration of the Sunset Assessment Scale, let's reflect on how this tool enhances our ability to make informed visit frequency decisions. This chapter shows how combining objective measurements with clinical judgment creates a more comprehensive patient assessment and care planning approach.

Key Takeaways

The Sunset Assessment Scale provides structure while honoring our clinical expertise. Remember Mrs. Thompson's case, where early recognition of declining scores enabled us to adjust visit frequencies proactively, supporting both patient and family through a challenging transition. Each scale component contributes to understanding patient needs while providing clear documentation to support our decisions.

Discussion Questions

1. Think about your most challenging patient case. How might applying the Sunset Assessment Scale have influenced your visit frequency decisions? What additional insights might it have provided?
2. Consider the clinical judgment modifier. When have you observed changes that weren't captured by standard assessments? How would this modifier have supported your decision-making?
3. How do you anticipate implementing this scale might change your current documentation practices? What benefits and challenges do you foresee?
4. Reflect on team communication. How might using this scale enhance your ability to justify visit frequency changes to your interdisciplinary team?

Practice Scenarios

Scenario 1: The New Admission

Mrs. Anderson, 82, was newly admitted with end-stage heart failure. Currently independent with ADLs but showing increasing fatigue. Eating 75% of meals, standard temperature patterns, occasional dyspnea with exertion.

- How would you score each component?
- What visit frequency would you recommend based on the total score?
- What changes would prompt you to use the clinical judgment modifier?

Scenario 2: The Changing Condition

Mr. Martinez has been on service for three months with end-stage COPD. The initial score was 14, but during today's visit, you note:

- Decreased activity tolerance
- Reduced appetite
- Normal temperature
- Increased work of breathing
- Family reporting increased anxiety
- Calculate his new score
- What changes would you make to visit frequency?
- How would you document your decision?

Scenario 3: The Complex Case

Mrs. Chen's physical scores remain stable at 12, but she shows increasing emotional distress, and family dynamics are strained. Her daughter reports difficulty managing medications.

- How would you apply the clinical judgment modifier?
- What visit frequency adjustments might be needed?
- How would you document your reasoning?

Moving Forward

As you integrate the Sunset Assessment Scale into your practice, remember that mastery comes through consistent application and reflection. Each patient offers opportunities to refine your assessment skills and deepen your understanding of this valuable tool.

Take time to practice scoring and documentation with your current patients. Share your experiences with colleagues and learn from their insights. Remember, excellence in hospice care requires both systematic assessment and clinical wisdom.

The skills we've explored in this chapter will serve as the foundation for even more sophisticated aspects of visit planning, which we'll discuss in upcoming chapters. Continue to grow in your practice, always keeping our ultimate goal in mind: providing the best possible care for our patients and families through well-planned, proactive visits.

Chapter 4: Comparative Analysis of Assessment Methods

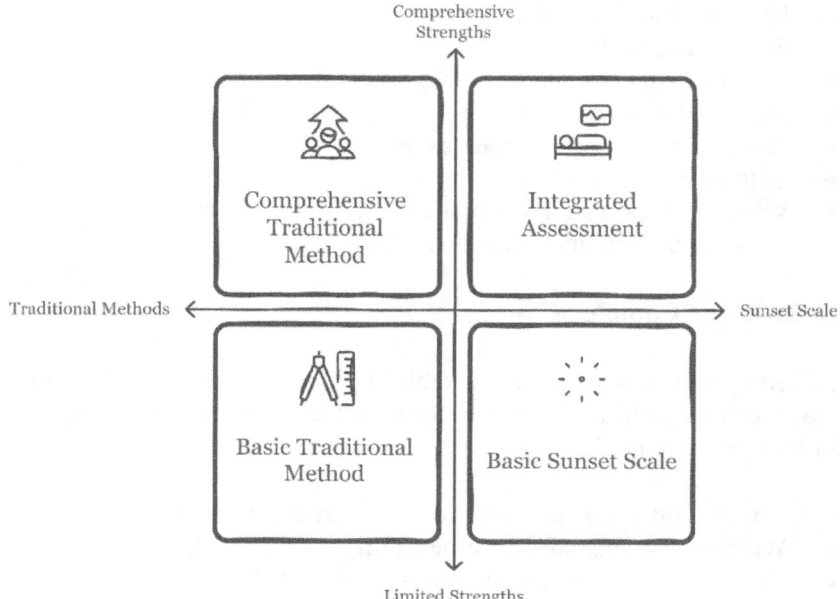

Throughout my career in hospice care, I've witnessed the evolution of assessment methods from simple checklists to sophisticated evaluation tools. Each advancement has brought new insights into determining visit frequencies and new implementation challenges. This chapter explores how traditional assessment methods and the Sunset Assessment Scale can enhance patient care.

When I first started in hospice, I relied primarily on the Palliative Performance Scale and basic symptom assessments. While these tools served us well, I often felt something was missing. Then, I met Mrs. Rodriguez, whose care taught me the value of combining different assessment approaches. Her case, which we'll explore in detail, demonstrates how integrating various tools can provide a more complete picture of patient needs.

Learning Objectives

After completing this chapter, you will be able to:

- Compare traditional assessment methods with the Sunset Assessment Scale
- Identify the unique strengths and limitations of different assessment approaches
- Develop effective strategies for integrating multiple assessment tools
- Implement best practices for assessment method adoption
- Apply combined assessment approaches to complex patient situations

Key Concepts

We'll begin by examining how traditional assessment methods and the Sunset Scale differ in their approaches to patient evaluation. Understanding these differences helps us recognize when each tool might be most valuable in our practice.

Next, we'll explore the strengths and limitations of various assessment methods. You'll learn how different tools complement each other, filling gaps that might exist when using any single approach alone.

We'll then delve into practical strategies for integrating multiple assessment methods into daily practice. Through real-world examples, you'll see how combining different approaches can enhance your ability to make informed visit frequency decisions.

Finally, we'll examine best practices for implementing new assessment methods in your organization. You'll learn from successful implementations and common pitfalls, helping you navigate the challenges of adopting new assessment tools.

Throughout this chapter, you'll meet patients like Mr. Thompson, whose complex symptoms required multiple assessment approaches, and Mrs. Chen, whose care demonstrated the value of integrated assessment methods. These cases will help you understand how to apply these concepts in your practice.

Remember, our goal isn't to replace one assessment method with another but to develop a comprehensive approach that enhances our ability to provide exceptional hospice care. Let's explore how we can combine traditional and new assessment methods to serve our patients and families better.

Traditional vs. Sunset Scale Approaches

Throughout my years in hospice care, I've used many assessment tools to guide visit frequency decisions. While traditional methods have served us well, introducing the Sunset Assessment Scale has transformed how we approach patient assessment. Let me share how these different approaches compare and complement each other.

I remember Mrs. Chen, an end-stage heart failure patient whose care taught me valuable lessons about assessment methods. Using traditional approaches, we relied heavily on the Palliative Performance Scale (PPS), which showed her at 60% - still relatively functional but requiring occasional assistance. While this provided helpful information about her physical status, it didn't fully capture her needs.

We gained additional insights when implementing the Sunset Assessment Scale with Mrs. Chen. Beyond measuring her functional status, we could systematically track her nutritional intake, temperature patterns, and breathing efforts. This comprehensive approach helped us identify subtle changes that might have gone unnoticed using traditional methods alone.

Traditional assessment methods often focus primarily on physical symptoms and functional status. While these remain crucial aspects of patient care, they sometimes miss the nuanced changes that signal the need for visit frequency adjustments. The PPS, for example, excels at measuring overall decline but may not capture the day-to-day variations that influence visit planning.

The Sunset Scale's strength lies in integrating multiple aspects of patient care while remaining simple for daily use. When Mr. Thompson's traditional assessments showed stable vital signs and pain levels, the Sunset Scale helped us identify increasing anxiety and subtle changes in his breathing patterns that warranted more frequent visits.

However, it's important to note that these approaches aren't mutually exclusive. The most effective patient care often combines traditional assessment methods with newer tools like the Sunset Scale. This integration allows us to maintain the validated reliability of traditional tools while benefiting from the more nuanced insights provided by the Sunset Scale.

Remember, our goal isn't to replace one assessment method with another but to use all available tools to provide the best possible care for our patients. Each approach offers unique insights that, when combined thoughtfully, enhance our ability to make informed visit frequency decisions.

Strengths and Limitations

Throughout my years in hospice care, I've learned that every assessment tool has unique strengths and limitations. Understanding these helps us choose the right approach for each situation while maintaining high-quality patient care.

Strengths of Traditional Tools

The Edmonton Symptom Assessment Scale (ESAS) has proven particularly valuable in my practice. I remember using it with Mr. Thompson, who struggled to communicate his symptoms. The ESAS helped identify his areas of concern and monitor changes over time. Its brevity and ease of use made it particularly effective during routine visits.

Traditional assessment tools also excel in providing standardized measurements that support quality monitoring across hospice organizations. They've been extensively validated and are widely accepted in palliative care settings. When Mrs. Chen's family questioned her declining condition, these objective measurements helped explain the changes we observed.

Limitations of Traditional Approaches

However, traditional tools sometimes fail to capture the whole picture. I've found that they often miss subtle changes that can signal the need for visit frequency adjustments. During my care for Mrs. Rodriguez, her standard assessments showed stable vital signs, but they didn't capture her increasing anxiety and family dynamics that warranted more frequent visits.

Another limitation I've encountered is the challenge of standardization. Despite explicit training, staff often struggle with who should be assessed and how frequently. This becomes particularly challenging with nonresponsive patients or those with severe dementia.

Strengths of the Sunset Scale

The Sunset Assessment Scale brings unique advantages to visit planning. Its comprehensive approach considers multiple aspects of patient care while remaining simple enough for daily use. When I started using it with Mr. Davis, I appreciated how it helped capture physical changes and subtle variations in his condition that might have gone unnoticed.

Limitations of Current Methods

One universal challenge across assessment tools is measuring the quality of care across different settings and populations. I've learned that no single tool perfectly addresses all aspects of hospice care. Some patients find numeric rating scales confusing, while others struggle with the formality of standardized assessments.

The key to successful assessment is combining different approaches while maintaining clinical judgment. Understanding these strengths and limitations allows us to select better and apply the right tools for each unique patient situation.

Integration Strategies

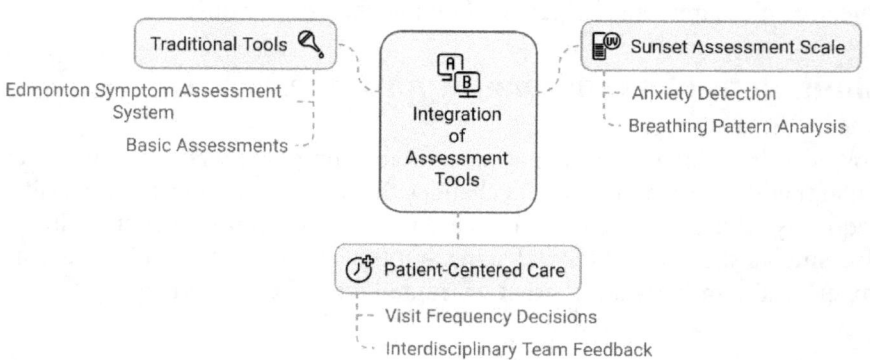

Throughout my years in hospice care, I've learned that successfully integrating different assessment methods requires a thoughtful, systematic approach. Let me share how we can effectively combine traditional tools with newer approaches like the Sunset Assessment Scale to create a more comprehensive care plan.

I remember working with Mrs. Rodriguez, whose complex symptoms challenged our traditional assessment methods. We understood her needs by integrating the Sunset Scale with our standard Edmonton Symptom Assessment System (ESAS). The ESAS helped us track her specific symptoms, while the Sunset Scale provided insights into subtle changes that influenced our visit frequency decisions.

The key to successful integration lies in understanding how different tools complement each other. For example, when Mr. Thompson's traditional assessments showed stable vital signs, the Sunset Scale helped us identify increasing anxiety and subtle changes in his breathing patterns that warranted more frequent visits. This combination of assessments provided more substantial documentation support for our care decisions.

One effective strategy I've found is to establish a systematic feedback process. When our interdisciplinary team began receiving regular updates combining both traditional and Sunset Scale assessments, we saw improved outcomes, particularly in managing depression and quality of life. This structured information-sharing approach helped ensure that all team members understood the rationale behind visit frequency changes.

Remember, integration isn't about using every available tool – it's about selecting and combining the right tools for each patient's unique situation. Sometimes, this means starting with basic assessments and gradually incorporating more sophisticated tools as we better understand the patient's needs.

The goal is to create a seamless assessment process that enhances our clinical judgment while maintaining the efficiency of our daily practice. When successfully integrating these tools, we're better equipped to provide proactive, patient-centered care that meets our patients' evolving needs.

Best Practices for Implementation

Throughout my years in hospice care, I've learned that successfully implementing new assessment methods requires careful planning and a supportive organizational culture. Let me share some proven strategies that have helped teams successfully integrate new assessment tools while maintaining quality patient care.

I remember when our hospice organization first implemented the Sunset Assessment Scale alongside our traditional tools. We started with Mrs. Chen's team—a small group of experienced nurses eager to enhance their practice. Their success taught us valuable lessons about effective implementation.

First, we learned the importance of leadership support. Our administrative team's visible commitment made a significant difference in staff acceptance. They didn't just announce the change; they provided resources, training time, and ongoing support throughout the implementation process.

The key to successful implementation lies in staff education and engagement. We found that nurses who understood how to use the tools and why they were valuable were likelier to embrace them. For example, when Mr. Thompson's nurse understood how combining traditional assessments with the Sunset Scale could provide earlier indicators of decline, she became one of our strongest advocates for the new approach.

Integrative Assessment Cycle

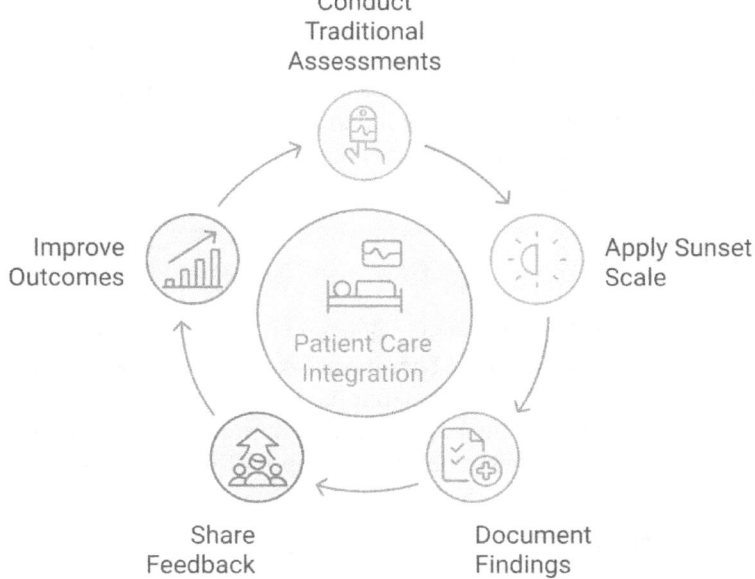

Another crucial element is creating a systematic feedback process. We established regular team meetings where nurses could share their experiences, challenges, and successes with the new assessment methods. This open dialogue helped us identify and address concerns early in the implementation process.

Remember to start small and build gradually. When implementing new assessment tools, begin with a pilot group of experienced nurses who can help refine the process before rolling it out to the entire organization. This approach allows you to address challenges on a smaller scale and build confidence in the new system.

Most importantly, the focus should be on patient outcomes. Regular monitoring of key indicators like symptom management effectiveness and family satisfaction helps demonstrate the value of new assessment methods while identifying areas needing adjustment.

Implementing new assessment methods takes time and patience. However, when done thoughtfully and with attention to these best practices, it can significantly enhance our ability to provide exceptional hospice care.

Conclusion to Chapter 4: Comparative Analysis of Assessment Methods

As we conclude our exploration of assessment methods, let's reflect on how combining different approaches enhances our ability to provide exceptional hospice care. This chapter shows how integrating traditional tools with the Sunset Assessment Scale creates a more comprehensive approach to patient evaluation and visit planning.

Key Takeaways

The art of assessment lies in knowing when and how to combine different tools effectively. Remember Mrs. Thompson's case, where traditional assessments showed stable vital signs, but the Sunset Scale revealed subtle changes that prompted early intervention. Each approach brings unique value to our practice, providing a more complete picture of our patients' needs.

Discussion Questions

1. Think about your current assessment practices. How might incorporating additional tools enhance your ability to determine appropriate visit frequencies? What challenges do you anticipate?
2. Consider a recent patient whose condition changed unexpectedly. What signs might you have caught earlier using a combination of assessment methods?
3. How do you currently document your rationale for visit frequency changes? How might integrating multiple assessment tools strengthen your documentation?
4. What strategies have you found effective when implementing new assessment methods in your practice? What lessons have you learned from less successful attempts?

Practice Scenarios

Scenario 1: The Complex Patient

Mrs. Anderson, 75, has end-stage COPD. Traditional assessments show stable vital signs and pain levels, but her daughter reports increasing anxiety and decreased appetite. Using both traditional tools and the Sunset Scale:

- How would you assess her current condition?
- What additional insights might each tool provide?
- How would you integrate these findings into your visit planning?

Scenario 2: The Implementation Challenge

Your hospice is introducing the Sunset Scale while maintaining traditional assessment methods. Some staff members express concern about "double documentation." Consider:

- How would you address these concerns?
- What implementation strategies might prove most effective?
- How would you demonstrate the value of integrated assessments?

Scenario 3: The Changing Condition

Mr. Martinez has been stable on weekly visits. His PPS score remains unchanged, but the Sunset Scale shows subtle changes in breathing patterns and activity levels.

- How would you reconcile these different findings?
- What additional assessments might be helpful?
- How would you adjust your visit frequency?

Moving Forward

As you integrate these assessment methods into your practice, remember that mastery comes through experience and reflection. Each patient offers opportunities to refine your assessment skills and deepen your understanding of how different tools complement each other.

Take time to practice combining assessment methods with your current patients. Share your experiences with colleagues and learn from their insights. Remember, excellence in hospice care requires both systematic assessment and clinical wisdom.

The skills we've explored in this chapter will serve as building blocks for even more sophisticated aspects of visit planning, which we'll discuss in upcoming chapters. Continue to grow in your practice, always keeping our ultimate goal in mind: providing the best possible care for our patients and families through well-planned, proactive visits guided by comprehensive assessment.

Chapter 5: Crisis Prevention Through Strategic PRN Planning

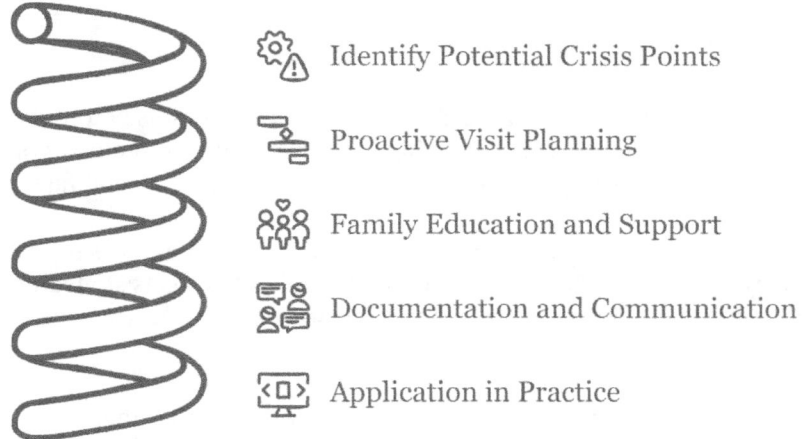

- Identify Potential Crisis Points
- Proactive Visit Planning
- Family Education and Support
- Documentation and Communication
- Application in Practice

Throughout my years in hospice care, I've learned that the most effective way to handle a crisis is to prevent it from happening. This chapter explores how strategic PRN visit planning can transform our practice from reactive to proactive care delivery, ultimately improving patient and family outcomes.

I remember my early days as a hospice nurse when I constantly responded to crisis calls. Then, I met Mrs. Thompson, whose case changed my perspective entirely. Her family called frequently about breakthrough pain, usually in the evenings. We dramatically reduced these crisis calls by implementing strategic PRN visits and family education while improving her symptom management. Her case, like many others we'll explore, demonstrates the power of preventive planning.

Learning Objectives

After completing this chapter, you will be able to:

- Recognize early warning signs that signal potential crisis points
- Develop strategic PRN visit plans that prevent common crisis situations

- Implement effective family education programs that build caregiver confidence
- Create documentation and communication protocols that support crisis prevention
- Transform reactive care patterns into proactive support systems

Key Concepts

We'll begin by exploring how to identify potential crisis points before they escalate into emergencies. Understanding these warning signs helps us plan interventions that prevent distressing situations for our patients and families.

Next, we'll examine proactive visit planning strategies that address needs before they become urgent. You'll learn to schedule PRN visits strategically, considering factors like symptom patterns, caregiver schedules, and support system availability.

We'll then delve into family education and support techniques that empower caregivers to manage situations confidently. Through real-world examples, you'll see how effective education reduces crisis calls while improving family satisfaction.

Finally, we'll explore documentation and communication protocols that enhance team coordination and support crisis prevention efforts. You'll learn how clear, specific documentation transforms our ability to provide proactive care.

Throughout this chapter, you'll meet patients like Mr. Rodriguez, whose evening pain crises were prevented through strategic PRN planning, and Mrs. Chen, whose family's confidence grew through targeted education and support. These cases will help you apply these concepts in your practice.

Remember, our goal isn't just to respond to crises – it's to prevent them through thoughtful planning and preparation. Let's explore how we can transform our approach to crisis prevention together.

Identifying Potential Crisis Points

Throughout my years in hospice care, I've learned that preventing crises often involves recognizing early warning signs and understanding common trigger points. Let me share how this knowledge has transformed my visit planning and crisis prevention approach.

I remember Mrs. Chen, a patient with end-stage COPD, whose daughter called our triage line frequently with anxiety about her mother's breathing. After analyzing these calls, I realized most occurred in the evening hours when her mother's dyspnea typically worsened. By scheduling a late afternoon PRN visit twice weekly, we prevented many of these crisis calls and provided better support for both patient and family.

Understanding crisis patterns helps us anticipate needs. Research shows that about 42% of hospice families experience what they perceive as a crisis during their hospice journey. These typically fall into three main categories: patient symptoms, emotional distress, and caregiver burden.

Let me tell you about Mr. Thompson, whose pain crisis taught me valuable lessons about prevention. His wife noticed his pain medications seemed less effective on Sundays - the day before his scheduled Monday visits. By identifying this pattern, we adjusted his visit schedule and implemented PRN visits on Sunday afternoons, preventing pain crises that had been occurring regularly.

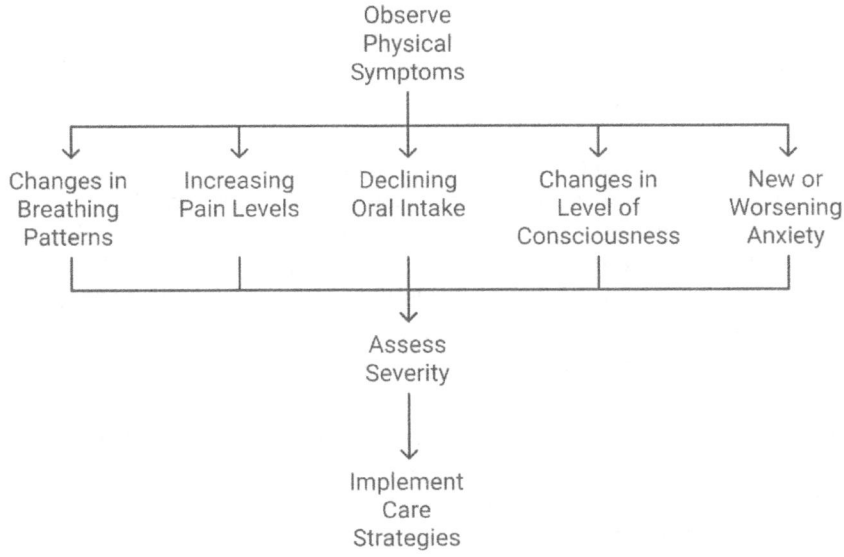

53 | **The Art of Hospice Visit Planning**

Physical symptoms often signal potential crisis points. Watch for the following:

- Changes in breathing patterns
- Increasing pain levels
- Declining oral intake
- Changes in the level of consciousness
- New or worsening anxiety

Caregiver burden represents another crucial area for crisis prevention. When Mrs. Rodriguez's daughter mentioned feeling overwhelmed with medication management, it signaled a potential crisis point. By scheduling PRN visits focused on medication teaching and support, we prevented medication errors and reduced caregiver stress.

Remember, many crises that appear suddenly actually show subtle warning signs days before. Recognizing these signs allows us to implement preventive measures through strategic PRN visit planning.

Proactive Visit Planning

Once we identify potential crisis points, the real art lies in planning visits that prevent these situations from developing. Throughout my career, I've learned that proactive visit planning isn't just about scheduling more visits – it's about scheduling the right visits at the right times.

Let me share a story about Mrs. Davis, a patient with end-stage heart failure. During routine visits, I noticed her anxiety increased significantly on weekends when her daughter worked. Instead of waiting for crisis calls, we scheduled PRN visits for Saturday mornings. These visits provided reassurance and symptom management before anxiety escalated into panic. This simple adjustment reduced after-hours calls by 80% and significantly improved patient and family satisfaction.

The key to proactive planning lies in understanding patterns. Consider Mr. Rodriguez's case. His pain typically worsened in the evenings, but our visits were scheduled for mornings. By adding a PRN visit in the late afternoon twice weekly, we could adjust his medication regimen before the pain escalated, preventing numerous crisis calls.

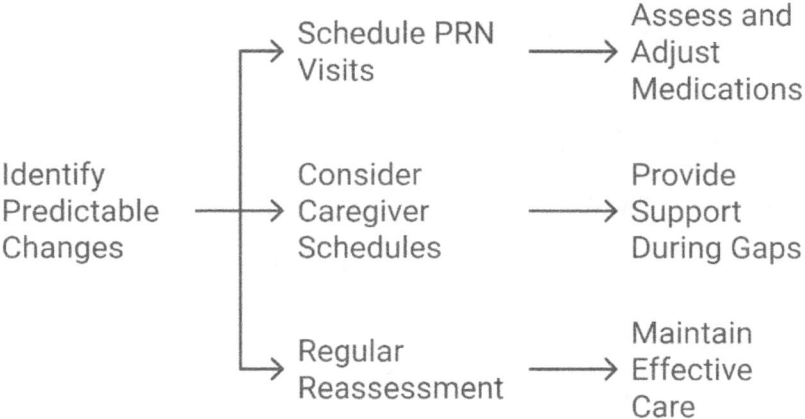

I've found that successful proactive visit planning involves several essential elements:

- First, we need to anticipate predictable changes. When Mrs. Thompson started showing signs of terminal restlessness in the evenings, we didn't wait for it to become a crisis. We scheduled PRN visits during early evening hours to assess and adjust medications before symptoms became severe.
- Second, we must consider caregiver schedules and support systems. One of my patients, Mr. Chen, had excellent family support except on Wednesdays when his primary caregiver attended church activities. By scheduling PRN visits during these times, we provided support when the family needed it most.
- Finally, remember that proactive planning requires regular reassessment. What works this week might need adjustment next week as conditions change. We can maintain effective crisis prevention while providing excellent care when we remain flexible and responsive to evolving needs.

The beauty of proactive visit planning lies in its ability to transform crisis-driven care into planned, systematic support. This approach improves patient care, reduces staff burnout, and improves overall hospice outcomes.

Remember, our goal isn't just to respond to crises – it's to prevent them through thoughtful, strategic visit planning that anticipates and addresses needs before they become emergencies.

Family Education and Support

Throughout my hospice career, I've learned that effective family education and support often differentiate between a well-managed situation and a crisis. Let me share how thoughtful family education transforms our ability to prevent crises through strategic PRN planning.

I remember Mrs. Thompson's family, particularly her daughter Sarah, who initially called our triage line multiple times weekly. Through targeted education and support, we helped Sarah understand the normal progression of her mother's heart failure and recognize early warning signs. More importantly, we taught her when to use PRN medications and when to request a PRN visit instead of waiting until the situation became urgent.

The key lies in making education practical and accessible. Consider Mr. Rodriguez's wife, Maria. Initially overwhelmed by medication management, she became confident after we created a simple medication calendar and practiced scenarios during our visits. We scheduled PRN visits specifically for medication teaching, which dramatically reduced her anxiety and prevented medication-related crises.

One approach that's proven particularly effective is what I call the "teach-back trilogy":

- First Visit: Introduce new concepts and demonstrate skills
- Second Visit: Have family practice while you observe
- Third Visit: Watch them perform tasks independently

Let me tell you about Mrs. Chen's family. During routine visits, we noticed they struggled with breakthrough pain management. Instead of just explaining the process, we scheduled three focused PRN visits:

- First visit: Demonstrated how to assess pain and administer PRN medications
- Second visit: Watched them perform an assessment and talk through medication decisions
- Third visit: Had them independently manage a pain episode while we provided support

This systematic approach to education transformed their confidence and significantly reduced crisis calls.

Remember, family education isn't just about teaching tasks – it's about empowering caregivers to feel confident in their roles. When we invest time in education during planned PRN visits, we create a foundation of understanding that prevents many potential crises.

The most successful family education programs include:

- Clear written instructions
- Practical demonstrations
- Regular practice opportunities
- Positive reinforcement
- Ongoing support and reassessment

By integrating education into our strategic PRN visit planning, we create a support system that helps families feel more confident and capable in their caregiving roles. This confidence often differentiates between a manageable situation and a perceived crisis.

Documentation and Communication Protocols

Throughout my years in hospice care, I've learned that effective documentation and communication protocols are essential for preventing crises and ensuring excellent patient care. Let me share how developing strong protocols has transformed my practice and improved outcomes for patients and families.

I remember Mrs. Chen's case, which taught me valuable lessons about documentation during crisis prevention. When we noticed her increasing anxiety in the evenings, we developed a specific documentation protocol for our PRN visits. Each note clearly outlined not just her symptoms but also our interventions and their effectiveness. This detailed documentation helped our entire team understand what approaches worked best, preventing future crises.

The key to effective crisis prevention documentation is "painting the picture" of what's happening with our patients. Rather than simply writing "anxiety increased," we document specific observations: what we see, hear, and measure. For example, with Mr. Thompson, we documented that the "respiratory rate increased from 20 to 28, visible shoulder tension, stating 'I can't catch my breath'" rather than just "breathing worse."

Communication protocols should focus on building trust through transparency and timeliness. When Mrs. Rodriguez's family expressed concerns about pain management, we implemented a communication protocol that included:

- Regular updates about medication effectiveness
- Clear documentation of family teaching
- Specific triggers for requesting PRN visits
- Written instructions for managing breakthrough symptoms

Remember to document both successful and unsuccessful interventions. This helps build a knowledge base for future crisis prevention. When documenting PRN visits, include:

- The specific trigger that prompted the visit
- Interventions attempted and their outcomes
- Family response and understanding
- Plan for follow-up

Effective protocols also include clear communication channels between team members. During Mrs. Davis's care, our team developed a system for sharing information about potential crisis points. Each discipline documented their observations using specific, measurable terms, allowing us to track patterns and prevent future crises.

Strong documentation and communication protocols are beautiful because they can transform reactive care into proactive support. Documenting thoroughly and communicating clearly creates a foundation for excellent crisis prevention and patient care.

Conclusion to Chapter 5: Crisis Prevention Through Strategic PRN Planning

As we conclude our exploration of crisis prevention through strategic PRN planning, let's reflect on how this proactive approach transforms patient care and family support. Throughout this chapter, we've seen how identifying potential crises early, planning preventive visits, effectively educating families, and maintaining clear communication can dramatically improve hospice outcomes.

Key Takeaways

The art of crisis prevention lies in anticipating needs before they become emergencies. Remember Mrs. Rodriguez's case, where strategic afternoon PRN visits prevented evening pain crises and reduced family anxiety? Each component we've discussed contributes to creating a comprehensive approach to crisis prevention that effectively serves patients and families.

Discussion Questions

1. Think about your most recent crisis call. What early warning signs might you have missed? How could strategic PRN planning have prevented this situation?
2. Consider your current approach to family education. How might incorporating the "teach-back trilogy" enhance your effectiveness in preventing crises?
3. What patterns do you notice in your after-hours calls? How could you use this information to plan preventive PRN visits?
4. How does your current documentation support or hinder crisis prevention? What changes might make it more effective?

Practice Scenarios

Scenario 1: The New Patient

Mrs. Anderson, newly admitted with end-stage COPD, lives with her daughter, who works evening shifts. Current symptoms include occasional dyspnea and anxiety, typically worsening in the evenings.

- How would you plan PRN visits to prevent crises?
- What family education would you prioritize?
- How would you document your prevention strategy?

Scenario 2: The Complex Family

Mr. Thompson receives excellent care from his wife, but she shows signs of caregiver fatigue. Their adult children visit regularly but seem uncertain about medication management.

- What potential crisis points do you identify?
- How would you structure family education?
- What PRN visit strategy would you implement?

Scenario 3: The Changing Condition

Mrs. Chen's symptoms have been well-managed with weekly visits, but she's showing early signs of decline. Her family expresses increasing anxiety about managing changes.

- How would you adjust your PRN visit planning?
- What education would help prevent crises?
- How would you document these changes?

Moving Forward

As you integrate these crisis prevention strategies into your practice, remember that success comes through consistent application and regular evaluation of outcomes. Each patient situation offers opportunities to refine your approach and deepen your understanding of effective crisis prevention.

Take time to analyze your current practices. Consider how you incorporate more strategic PRN planning into your daily work. Share your insights with colleagues and learn from their experiences. Remember, excellence in hospice care requires both proactive planning and responsive care.

The skills we've explored in this chapter will serve as the foundation for providing exceptional hospice care that truly meets the needs of our patients and families. Continue to grow in your practice, always keeping our ultimate goal in mind: providing comprehensive, proactive care that prevents crises while supporting patients and families through their hospice journey.

Conclusion

As we conclude our journey through the art of hospice visit planning, I'm reminded of why we chose this challenging yet rewarding field. Throughout my career, I've witnessed how thoughtful visit planning transforms patient care and entire family experiences during the hospice journey.

Call to Action for Excellence

The future of hospice care lies in our hands. Every visit we plan, every assessment we complete, and every family we educate shape the quality of end-of-life care in our communities. Mrs. Thompson's daughter told me, "Your careful planning made all the difference in Mom's final weeks." These moments remind us why excellence in visit planning matters so profoundly.

We must commit to continuous improvement in our practice. This means regularly evaluating our visit planning strategies, embracing new assessment tools, and seeking ways to serve our patients and families better. The Sunset Assessment Scale and strategic PRN planning are just the beginning—our field continues to evolve, and we must evolve with it.

Future Directions in Visit Planning

The landscape of hospice care is changing rapidly. Telehealth visits, remote monitoring, and artificial intelligence are becoming integral parts of our practice. I recently worked with Mr. Rodriguez's family, using a combination of in-person and virtual visits to provide more frequent support without overwhelming their daily routine. This blended approach represents just one way our field is adapting to meet changing needs.

We're seeing emerging trends in:

- Predictive analytics for crisis prevention
- Mobile documentation solutions
- Integration of family feedback systems
- Enhanced communication platforms

Resources for Continued Learning

Excellence requires ongoing education. I encourage you to:

- Join professional hospice organizations
- Participate in continuing education programs
- Engage in peer learning groups
- Study quality improvement methodologies
- Share your own experiences and insights

Quality Improvement Strategies

Quality improvement in visit planning isn't just about meeting metrics—it's about enhancing the care we provide. Consider starting with small changes, like implementing the Sunset Assessment Scale with one patient, and then expanding based on what you learn. When our team began tracking crisis calls in relation to visit patterns, we discovered opportunities for improvement we hadn't previously recognized.

Remember Mrs. Chen's case? Our quality improvement efforts led us to develop better family education protocols, resulting in fewer crisis calls and higher family satisfaction scores. Each slight improvement contributes to better patient care.

As we close this book, I challenge each of you to implement one concept you've learned in your practice this week. Whether using a new assessment tool, planning strategic PRN visits, or enhancing your documentation protocols, every step toward improvement matters.

The art of hospice visit planning continues to evolve, but our core mission remains constant: providing exceptional end-of-life care that honors our patients and supports their families. Together, we can elevate the standard of hospice care through thoughtful, strategic visit planning.

Remember, excellence in hospice care isn't a destination – it's a journey of continuous learning and improvement. Let's continue this journey together, always striving to provide the best possible care for our patients and families.

Resources and References

Hospice Nursing Visit Frequencies: A Guide for New Hospice Nurses at https://compassioncrossing.info/nursing-visit-frequencies-on-hospice-a-guide-for-new-hospice-nurses/

Considerations for Increasing Hospice Visit Frequencies at https://compassioncrossing.info/considerations-for-increasing-hospice-visit-frequencies/

The Sunset Assessment Scale for Determining Hospice Skilled Nursing Visit Frequencies at https://compassioncrossing.info/the-sunset-assessment-scale-for-determining-hospice-skilled-nursing-visit-frequencies/

Exploring the Association of Hospice Care on Patient Experience and Outcomes of Care at https://pmc.ncbi.nlm.nih.gov/articles/PMC5313381/

Hospice Care Linked to Higher Family Satisfaction at https://www.oldcolonyhospice.org/blog/hospice-care-linked-to-higher-family-satisfaction

The Value of Hospice Care: Hospice Utilization and the Importance of Referring Your Patient Early at https://www.vnshealth.org/for-professionals/insights/the-value-of-hospice-care-hospice-utilization-and-the-importance-of-referring-your-patient-early/

How to achieve compliance in hospice care plans at https://www.citushealth.com/blog/how-to-achieve-adherence-and-compliance-to-hospice-care-plans/

Barriers Faced by Healthcare Providers during Home Visits of Palliative Care Patients – A Qualitative Study at https://pmc.ncbi.nlm.nih.gov/articles/PMC11021074/

Shared decision making in-home hospice nursing visits: A qualitative study at https://pmc.ncbi.nlm.nih.gov/articles/PMC6335643/

Assessment Tools for Palliative Care at in-home at https://effectivehealthcare.ahrq.gov/sites/default/files/pdf/palliative-care-tools_technical-brief-2017.pdf

Prognostication and Scoring Tools at https://www.compassus.com/healthcare-professionals/prognostication-scoring-tools/

National Palliative Care Research Center Measurement and Evaluation Tools at http://www.npcrc.org/content/25/measurement-and-evaluation-tools.aspx

Understanding Changes in Palliative Performance Scale in the Last Six Months of Life at https://compassioncrossing.info/understanding-changes-in-palliative-performance-scale-in-the-last-six-months-of-life/

Understanding Functional Decline in the Natural Dying Process at https://compassioncrossing.info/understanding-functional-decline-in-the-natural-dying-process/

Frequency of Changes in Condition as an Indicator of Approaching Death at https://compassioncrossing.info/velocity-of-changes-in-condition-as-an-indicator-of-approaching-death/

Understanding Terminal Illness Progression: Observable Signs and Symptoms at https://compassioncrossing.info/understanding-terminal-illness-progression-observable-signs-and-symptoms/

Sleeping as a Prognostication Tool for the Terminally Ill at https://compassioncrossing.info/sleeping-as-a-prognostication-tool-for-the-terminally-ill/

Kindred at Home Hospice Eligibility Documentation Tips and Strategies 2 at https://s3.amazonaws.com/GentivaUniversity/JobAids/Hospice+Eligibility+Documentation+Tips+and+Strategies.pdf

Hospice Documentation at https://www.cgsmedicare.com/hhh/coverage/coverage_guidelines/hospice_documentation.html

Receipt of Hospice Aide Visits Among Medicare Beneficiaries Receiving Home Hospice Care at https://pmc.ncbi.nlm.nih.gov/articles/PMC8930441/

Top Indicators for the Hospice Care Index at https://hospice.eewebinarnetwork.com/Top-Indicators-for-the-Hospice-Care-Index

Opening the Envelope: Understanding the Hospice Care Index Inaugural Report at https://activatedinsights.com/articles/opening-the-envelope-understanding-the-hospice-care-index-inaugural-report/

Pre-Visit Planning: Save Time, Improve Care, and Strengthen Care Team Satisfaction at https://edhub.ama-assn.org/steps-forward/module/2702514

Best Practices For Hospice Team Collaboration at https://www.eminencehhcma.com/blog/best-practices-for-coordinating-care-within-a-hospice-team

Enhancing Patient Communication in Hospice at https://www.breezehospiceservices.com/resources/enhancing-patient-communication-in-hospice

Improving Hospice Outcomes through Systematic Assessment: A Clinical Trial at https://pmc.ncbi.nlm.nih.gov/articles/PMC3036771/

Use These Medicare Assessments for Hospice Eligibility at https://www.axxess.com/blog/regulatory/use-these-medicare-assessments-for-hospice-eligibility/

CMS CAHPS® Hospice Survey at https://www.cms.gov/medicare/quality/hospice/cahpsr-hospice-survey

Perceptions of a Home Hospice Crisis: An Exploratory Study of Family Caregivers at https://pmc.ncbi.nlm.nih.gov/articles/PMC6735312/

Contingency and Crisis Standards of Care – Palliative Care and Hospice Services at https://www.nationalhospiceanalytics.com/library/CSC/1_Crisis_Standards_of_Care_-_Palliative_Care__Hospice_-_final_06.19.20.pdf

Best Practices in End of Life and Palliative Care in the Emergency Department at https://pmc.ncbi.nlm.nih.gov/articles/PMC11300921/

Communication between healthcare professionals and relatives of patients approaching the end-of-life: A systematic review of qualitative evidence at https://pmc.ncbi.nlm.nih.gov/articles/PMC6691601/

End-of-life communication strategies for healthcare professionals: A scoping review at https://journals.sagepub.com/doi/full/10.1177/02692163221133670

State Operations Manual Appendix M - Guidance to Surveyors: Hospice at https://www.cms.gov/Regulations-and-Guidance/Guidance/Manuals/downloads/som107ap_m_hospice.pdf

Author Bio

Peter Abraham, BSN, RN is an experienced nurse dedicated to supporting nurses, caregivers, families, and patients in their learning, growth, and well-being journey. Peter's nursing path encompasses practical experience as a cardiac telemetry nurse in a bustling cardiology unit at a Magnet-awarded teaching hospital. Additionally, Peter has fulfilled the role of a second-shift RN supervisor, overseeing an entire building in an SNF/LTC (Skilled Nursing Facility/Long-Term Care) setting with 151 residents. Remarkably, during the initial wave of COVID-19, the facility achieved an impressive close-to-100% recovery rate before operation warp speed was complete.

Furthermore, Peter's nursing career extends to rural home hospice care. As a visiting hospice registered nurse case manager, he offers compassionate care to patients in various settings, including private homes, personal care homes, assisted living facilities, skilled nursing facilities, and hospitals.

Moreover, Peter's desire to help others extends beyond his physical presence. At CompassionCrossing.Info, he writes articles to empower caregivers, family members, and fellow nurses in end-of-life care. Peter's drive to help others, which flows from his love of Christ Jesus, is a source of support and encouragement for all he reaches.

Other books by Peter Abraham include the following:

Empowering Excellence in Hospice: A Nurse's Toolkit for Best Practices series:

> Compliance-based, Eligibility Driven Hospice Documentation: Tips for Hospice Nurses
> Whispers of Time: Understanding the End-of-Life Timeline
> Mastering Hospice Eligibility: An Essential Guide for RNs and Clinical Managers
> Mastering Recertifications: A Comprehensive Guide for Nurses
> Conversations at the End: Guiding Families Through Final Days
> Mastering the Hospice Item Set: A Comprehensive Guide for Nurses and Managers
> Care Plans for Hospice Patients: A Comprehensive Guide
> Mindful Minutes: Time Management Secrets for Hospice Nursing Excellence
> Medication Reconciliation in Hospice Care: Maximizing Quality of Life
> HOPE in Practice: Implementing Patient-Centered Outcomes in Hospice Care
> The Complete Hospice Visit: A Nurse's Guide to Excellence
> The Art of Hospice Visit Planning: A Clinical Guide to Patient-Centered Care Frequency

Compassionate Caregiving series:

> Daily Hospice Care Planner: Organize, Communicate, and Provide Consistent Care
> Dignity in Dying: A Thoughtful Approach to Voluntary Stopping Eating and Drinking
> Palliative Sedation: A Compassionate Approach
> Hospice Medication Handbook: A Caregiver's Guide to Comfort Medications
> Nourishing Hope: A Caregiver's Guide to End-of-Life Nutrition
> Validation and Compassion: A Guide to Connecting with Terminally Ill Loved Ones
> Palliative Care vs Hospice Care: Making Informed Decisions
> Understanding Your Rights in Hospice Care: A Guide for Patients and Families

When It's Time for Hospice: A Compassionate Guide for Families and Caregivers
The Caregiver's Lifeline: Self-Care in End-of-Life Care

Dementia Caregivers Essentials series:

Dementia Caregiver Essentials (all ten books below in one)

Anger Management in Dementia
CPAP and Oxygen for Dementia
Diabetes Care for Dementia
Hallucination Management for Dementia
Infection Awareness in Dementia
Medication Compliance for Dementia
Music Therapy for Dementia
Nutrition for Dementia
Placement for Dementia
Sundowning Management for Dementia

Holistic Nurse: Skills for Excellence series

Compassionate Care in Conflict: A Nurse's Guide to Managing Combative Patients
Dementia Staging Mastery: A Nurse's Guide to Dementia Assessment
The Nurse's Guide to Motivational Interviewing: Empowering Patients to Make Lasting Health Changes

The above books can be found on Amazon at https://amzn.to/3YFBYQ0

Connect with Peter On:

Website: https://compassioncrossing.info/

www.ingramcontent.com/pod-product-compliance
Lightning Source LLC
Chambersburg PA
CBHW070402230526
45471CB00006B/2664